The Biochemical Key

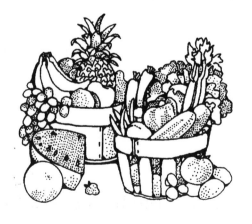

Barbara Schipper-Bergstein

The Biochemical Key

A practical way to control your weight - advice and recipes

Astrolog Publishing House

Astrolog Publishing House
P. O. Box 1123, Hod Hasharon 45111, Israel
Tel: 972-9-7412044
Fax: 972-9-7442714
E-Mail: info@astrolog.co.il
Astrolog Web Site: www.astrolog.co.il

Astrolog Publishing House © 2002

ISBN 965-494-128-7

Published by Astrolog Publishing House 2002

Printed in Israel
1 3 5 7 9 10 8 6 4 2

Contents

What it's all about

The fact that we're happy to accept good things that come our way is not surprising. But how is it that we also tend to accept things that aren't pleasant? For example, we look in the mirror every day, and the image there tells us that our clothes don't fit the way they did when we first bought them, and our profile has turned into a thicker shape. Not pleasant! We tend to ignore what we think we can get away with.

Going out to meet the day pulls our thoughts away from being heavy and anyway, tomorrow we can check again in the mirror to see if something really has to be done about the extra weight. So we accept this undesirable development without being aware that we're doing so. In time, we find that our energy level has dropped silently and unnoticed, until we begin to feel tired when doing things that never required much effort in the past. This unexpected, unwanted and strange difference in our body can happen at any age. It normally creeps up slowly, quietly, but definitely, and soon we decide that the feeling of tightness at the waist is just too uncomfortable to bear. So we gradually replace our clothing with a larger size, until we need yet a larger size. As our silhouette swells, we begin to make adjustments in our movements to comply with the smaller amount of energy that has become available.

We accept this gentle downhill slope as a natural side effect of being an adult - don't most adults get heavier, fatter, we think as we look around at others? The once fresh, thin, healthy person is gradually nowhere to be found in the mirror, which instead reflects a tired and overweight figure. Almost without fail, we reach a point - and this generally repeats itself in a cyclical manner - when we say to ourselves, "That's it. I look terrible. I must do something about my weight." This mantra is followed by diets that are found in advertisements, recommended by friends, or referred by a doctor - or some self-conceived strategy that logic has contrived.

Optimism is a great motivator to get us on to the road to looking great again. With all the excitement of a clever decision to join a weight loss group, or buy magic weight-loss pills and potions, we begin with all the seriousness of a determined effort to change our eating habits.

Soon, the great new hope of being slim begins to fade. It feels unreachable, the effort becomes too great, and the outcome is already beginning to spell failure!

Nevertheless, almost like routine, the cycle repeats itself: dieting is a must, changed eating habits again bring some results, but then the struggle with hunger becomes painfully frustrating, the temptation of forbidden foods overcomes the will to continue, the diet is dropped and weight is regained, reaching yet a higher level. Soon, you'll be ready for the next round. This pattern is known as yoyo dieting. It's a game of slimming down and puffing up - "slim and puff, slim and puff," and with each puff, the pot(belly) gets bigger.

Seeing the high number of voluminous people who stick out in a crowd is testimony to the fact that obesity has reached epidemic proportions in the U.S. and threatens developed societies everywhere. It provides evidence of the many failed attempts to lose weight.

I was shocked to find that I was actually moving in that direction. How could gradual change in my own self have any shock value? How could I not see it coming? The answer is that it can indeed happen. We tend to accept changes that are dictated by time as though they are inevitable, probably because what is brought on by a natural factor such as time is considered to be inevitable. But it's not, I later learned!

Reflections about myself led to questions that brought eye-opening discoveries. The first one came from lab tests. Despite my futile efforts to keep thin, I looked puffy. I wasn't seriously overweight, but my face and neck had lost their sharp contours, my middle protruded more, and trying to avoid becoming seriously overweight, I had reduced my food intake to one meager meal a day. I was able to deal with between-meal hunger with snacks of chocolate, more than the occasional helping of ice-cream, and of course my favorite, potato chips - until I discovered that I was actually slowly killing myself. This emerged from a routine visit to my doctor when he told me that my cholesterol was beginning to reach the danger level. He took my blood pressure and said that it was too high to ignore. After a period of monitoring, he decided that I would have to go on medication. I reacted with dread when I was told that the treatment to lower blood pressure is a lifelong matter.

This came as a shock. My mind raced through an imagined scenario - take the pills and suffer side effects then take medication to deal with the side effects, then feel the loss of spontaneity that prescription drugs tend to produce and then take medicine to help pick me up. In short, this was the beginning of the end of the person I knew, the self that I thought I valued and imagined that I had looked after so well.

At first I resisted, arguing that medication was not going to help me in the long run. I was angry, I felt helpless, and I was definitely not going to start a parade of visits between the doctor and the pharmacy on a regular basis to monitor the medication. I was sure about that.

Until I was told that high blood pressure was a silent killer.

I knew that I was especially vulnerable because of the strong prevalence of heart disease in my family. My father and his brothers died of coronary disease in their forties.

So my anger subsided, and in its place came the fear of you-know-what. That was when I decided to go along with the doctor's recommendation. With no other choice, I agreed to take medication, but not without a very strong determination to try to lick this some other way. I set my mind to seeking a less intimidating solution. I decided to look for a way to reclaim my good health naturally, a way that would help me stop the medication.

The first thing I learned was that my doctor didn't share my concern about a lifetime of medication. His approach was to treat the symptoms while ignoring the causes that lay at the root of my medical problem. He felt confident about the prognosis. With medication, my blood pressure would go down and this would reduce the probability of heart disease. I, on the other hand, was convinced that the issue was not closed.

And so I took stock of my self. I found that beyond being chubby, there was a list of unwelcome developments that were affecting my health so innocently that they were barely noticeable. I noticed that my lower legs were puffy and that my ankles, once slender, were no longer visible. Well, that may be part of normal development, I thought. As we develop we grow, don't we? After all, this has been happening to us since childhood. It was at this point that reality splashed over me like a cold shower.

I soon found myself in the first round of the slim and puff game - but I was looking for a way to stop the game on the slim side. I couldn't stop eating chocolate, and that brought me to the realization that I had developed a craving for it. My passion for potatoes in any shape or form was not a helpful habit. Also, eating one meal a day was frustrating because it wasn't controlling my weight. Even at this one and only meal of the day I would try to control the amount I should be eating. I also noticed that when I felt hungry, my moods were unstable, and I became irritable for no reason. Trivial issues were enough to bring on little nervous tensions. It also seemed that I was fighting hunger all the time.

I decided to survey the literature about the causes of high cholesterol and blood pressure, and learn about the latest developments in healthy eating. I set myself the task of reading whatever information I could find that had become available over the past two decades. For months I read and collected information from articles, books, and the Internet. I soon discovered that an entire school of nourishment had emerged that is being referred to as the "new nutrition." It is an approach that is slowly replacing traditional calorie diets that served as the standard recommendation for weight loss since the early years of the 20th century. Following almost universal failure, calorie counting for menu building is now being recognized as a weak and ineffective method for losing weight. This is one of the villains that fuels the slim and puff game!

After months of study, I decided to change my eating habits. I am now thinner and healthier. I eat three to five times more than ever, and I was able to reduce the dose of medication because my blood pressure is normal! What disturbs me medically (because I didn't receive counseling from my doctor) and morally (because it's a doctor's duty to guide his patients to health) is that I had to do this on my own. I had to find my own way because the medical community, it seems, is traditionally bound to prescribing medication to reduce symptoms, which may be an honorable pursuit, but it doesn't always get to the root of the problem. The new nutrition, however, deals with the *causes* of high blood pressure, high cholesterol, and type II diabetes, not only their symptoms. It seems that medical doctors, for the most part, are reluctant to use the principles of correct nutrition that emerged from many clinical studies that have been accumulating since the 1980s.

Compiled from the latest studies, the book you are holding explains why the calorie method for losing weight doesn't succeed; why you gain weight; how blood pressure, cholesterol, and adult onset diabetes are related; why you get hungry long before the next meal; and how to lose weight. In summary, a clear understanding of the "new nutrition" can put you in complete control of your nutritional health.

You may decide that eating ice cream, cake and chips is more important to you than making an effort to become healthy. BUT, after reading this book you will know how you can lose weight if you should decide (not only want) to. You may rightly ask why you should believe what you'll read here. The simple truth is that the information contained here is correct and authentic because it has been collected from tested and published results. The explanation of weight control that you will read here is taken from scientific and medical sources that explain the reasons for your excess weight and how the body reacts to different food categories. You will understand clearly why the

Biochemical Key method is effective, and why following it will guide you back to good health. You will learn the reasons for weight gain, what to eat that actually helps you lose weight, and how to set out on the path to feeling great.

Apart from my own weight loss success, working with people who needed to reduce their weight has been exceedingly gratifying. If I live to a ripe old age and in good health, it will be due to the blessings that they showered upon me. Some wrote letters:

> **Dear Barbara,**
>
> *My wife says that because of you and your wonderful meal management method, she has fallen in love with me all over again.*
>
> *Over the last several years I have been progressively and constantly gaining weight. All my attempts to lose weight and the ugly stomach that came along with it failed. Diets of all types as well as walking and exercise did nothing much to alleviate the situation. Now I am told by people who haven't seen me for several months that I look like I used to look years ago. Friends who I haven't seen for a long time stop me on the street and tactfully ask what happened to me because I'm so much thinner. I have lost seven kilos, but because of the natural and unique process of weight redistribution I look like I have lost much more. The only disadvantage is that I have had to alter or give away my trousers,*

which have become miles too big for me. Thank you for returning my original figure to me.

Danny L.

Dear Barbara,
When you told me about the Biochemical Key, the things you said were hard to believe. But they are all true. For the first time in my life I am eating three healthy meals a day, consuming huge quantities of food and losing weight. The best part of it is that the weight is being redistributed in my body so that slimming is occurring in formerly problematic areas such as under my chin, my buttocks and my stomach. My lifelong tiredness and moodiness have disappeared. I feel energetic and look, I am told, better than ever! After approximately three weeks on the Biochemical Key method, I began to suffer from tremendous exhaustion (which can happen due to the change in diet, as you had said). Blood test results were normal, so I continued. This lasted far into the second month.
Now I feel fantastic. I have discovered a new hobby - and that is eating! For an entire lifetime I have been eliminating and reducing types and amounts of food due to my tendency to gain weight. Now the more I eat, the more I lose. This is of course

*entirely without any form of pills or medication, but
with strict adherence to what I eat.
Tell people : Do you want another chance? - DO IT!
You'll never regret it.
Thank you, Barbara, you saved my life.*

Ada

Dear Barb,
*It works!
I have lost close to 20 lbs. I eat well and am not
finding the diet restrictive although I love potatoes,
white bread and have a nasty sweet tooth. Even
though the weight doesn't come off as fast as I
would like, I persevere because I am feeling well
and I feel better about myself. I don't bulge out of
my clothes and I fit into my wardrobe. The best part
is I don't snack anymore because I don't crave it the
way I used to. And I don't feel stuffed anymore
after a hearty meal. It's a good way of eating well
and losing weight, too.*

Bayla R.

Exploding the diet myths

If the following describes you, you're probably an experienced dieter in search of a plan that works:

You find it hard to stop eating bread, pasta, sweets once you've started.

You find yourself getting hungry soon after a meal.

You try to control what you eat but you find yourself giving up because you're craving for food.

There are as many diets on the market as there are people with ideas to sell. What this indicates is that when there are many ways to solve an uncomplicated problem, it is surely because a valid, effective method hasn't been found, and this is true of weight control - until now, that is.

Has it ever occurred to you to ask why so many methods are recommended? The fact is that for the most part they don't produce the results that they are expected to deliver. When this happens, you're led to believe it's your fault. In their book, *The Carbohydrate Addict's Diet*, Drs. Rachael and Richard Heller wrote this dedication: "To the untold numbers of carbohydrate addicts who, deep down, have always known that it was not their fault."

After all, you were convinced that the diet worked for others, which convinced you that you should look to yourself for the reason for failure. You believe that if the diet didn't work for you, it's because you're weak-willed, you don't have the power to resist temptation, and at some point you'll start again - only this time, you'll try harder. Then, when you fail again, your self-criticism grows, you find yourself agonizing over your inability to stick to it, and you may begin to succumb to what has become your most profound pleasure in life, which is eating. At this point, the "slim and puff" game is over, and you lost on the puffy side.

This pattern is not as predetermined as you might think. In fact, it's not the only route, and you're about to learn the reason why. Many people have told me that when they lost weight, they lived in fear of putting it back on. They were caught in an almost obsessive situation because they felt that they were holding on precariously to their lower weight, without any sense of control. What they were saying was that they didn't know how to take charge of their eating in order to maintain the success they had worked so hard to achieve. They felt they would be unable to resist the temptations that always ended their previous attempts to lose weight.

You're likely to be shocked by what you read here because I'm going to challenge everything you were told about how you should eat to lose weight. You'll understand for the first time why all your past attempts failed; why you find it hard to stop eating (it's not because of weak will power); why overeating is not the real demon, and what you must eat to lose weight.

Many people lose a lot of weight. One of my colleagues,

who was a slim and puff player for many years, used to say that he had lost 2,000 pounds - he didn't mention over how many years! The success rate for long-term maintenance of weight loss with traditional diets is reported to be less than 5%. This means that almost everyone regains their lost weight, and often even more, within one year. This success rate is lower than programs that are designed to help people quit smoking or stop the excessive use of alcohol, which have success rates that are more than double that figure. So, 5% succeed on low-calorie diets, while on methods that are based on the new nutrition, the success rate is reported to be over 75%.

After countless serious efforts to lose weight fails, frustration accumulates and lowers our confidence that any effort could lead to success. Most people who have tried to diet can describe their long and sorry history of disappointment that increases with each failure. This leads to the loss of hope of ever gaining control of their weight, and reduces their belief in the concept of dieting. What's more, the dieters themselves are usually blamed, and willingly take the blame for their failures. Their experience has taught them that diets don't do what they're supposed to.

Calorie traditionalists advise dieters to eat low calorie food and snacks such as dry rice cakes and popcorn, claiming that the weight is gained from the cream or butter or jam that is put on them - not true, as you'll soon discover. They advise hungry dieters to relieve their empty feeling with fresh vegetables, when everyone knows that vegetables are simply unsatisfying because they don't have the capacity to reduce hunger.

The new nutrition, which is also referred to as the hormonal approach to healthy eating and weight control, is revolutionary because it rejects the norms that were established years ago for good nutrition, and replaces them with an effective program of meal management. It isn't a diet. It may have a date to mark the beginning, but managing meals correctly is essential for a healthy life, and lasts as long.

The following food pyramid that was in our schools' health textbooks decades ago continues to be promoted by health authorities today. It looks like this. (The idea of the pyramid means you're to eat the smallest amounts of the food groups that appear at the top of the pyramid, and as the pyramid expands, to eat more of the food that appears on the lower lines, and finally, to eat the largest amount of the food group that appears at the bottom.)

> *...Fat & sweets...*
> *.....Dairy & protein.....*
> *.....Fruits and vegetables.....*
> *............Carbohydrates............*

The new nutrition endorses a different food pyramid that looks like this:

...Carbs/starches...
.....Unsaturated fat.....
.............Fruits.............
.........Low -fat protein........
..............Vegetables...............

The first pyramid is a confirmed prescription for gaining weight. The second pyramid is a program for good nutrition. But since it is still the "new boy on the block," it is not yet being endorsed by most physicians, nor are they appreciated by them - probably because they have not taken the time to study the merits of the new nutrition.

We're all victims of the media that pound away at us by attractively packaged advertisements, reports of diet fads, and processed foods. We're also led to believe that obesity is an inherent condition that causes us to overeat. What is closer to the truth is that at most, seriously overweight people may have a stronger tendency to produce and store fat, but they've been following the first pyramid and eating the wrong food for a long time, and this is what led to their weight problem. Obesity is a condition that is caused by an addiction, and not - as it is believed - by the amounts that they eat. We now know that while certain foods can bring on hunger, other foods are very satisfying and take a long time to digest. From this we've learned that weight loss can be promoted by eating certain foods. These important facts are among the scientific findings that you'll discover further on.

We've been told again and again that counting calories is the correct method for losing weight. This misleading notion is perpetuated despite its failure. And because we're led to believe that the method is correct and we're doing something wrong, we try to follow a low-calorie diet again and again without much long-term success. The fact is that a low-calorie diet fails to produce a feeling of satisfaction, and it does not provide us with the type of food that will prevent us from feeling hungry between meals.

This is how the misleading calorie principle was born. In the 1930s, two American doctors suggested that a high-calorie diet will cause unexpended calories to be stored as fat, which is how we gain weight. So if you're accustomed to eating 2,500 calories and you decide to diet and reduce your calorie intake to only 2,000 calories, the doctors suggested that this would create a calorie deficit and as a consequence you would lose weight. The reverse would also be true. According to them, a 3,500 daily calorie intake would produce an increase in weight because the extra 1,000 calories would be stored as fat. This theory seemed rational and was adopted by the medical profession. Unfortunately, it is not totally correct.

This is because their research was incomplete. We know that the body reacts to the lower intake of calories by shedding weight. But now, after all these years we have learned that the calorie method can sustain weight loss only in the short term. What was not taken into account in the past when the calorie method was being researched was the body's inclination to adjust itself to a lower calorie intake. So in fact, the body's adjustment to the lower calorie amount causes it to burn less than the 2,000 that it has become accustomed to, and will store the remainder as fat. This indicates that the dieting equation according to the calorie theory is invalid because of the body's tendency to adjust to its new output of energy, which is less when we weigh less! It's simply a matter of realizing that a lighter body will burn less energy! Eating fewer calories doesn't contribute to genuine, long-term weight loss because the biochemical process will actually cause the body to resist. So, the less you weigh, the lower your calorie intake must be in order to continue losing weight. And, on a practical level, eating fewer calories is less satisfying.

In light of this information, calorie planning should be discarded and replaced by hormonal planning. To do this, we are turning the U.S. government's directive to follow the low fat / high cholesterol pyramid upside down, and instead recommending a balanced diet that consists of high fiber / low carbohydrates / unsaturated fat / low-fat protein, which will be described.

The hormonal approach or new nutrition started with researchers, many of whom had a weight problem themselves. For example, Michel Montignac, who began writing about the causes of obesity in the 1980s, tells his story in his book, *Eat Yourself Slim*: When he was a young boy, he was already heavier than his friends. As with most growing boys, he slimmed down to normal during his adolescence. About ten years later he started to struggle with his weight again. From then on, he was constantly preoccupied with trying to keep his weight down. Despite all his efforts, he found himself more seriously overweight when he was nearing middle age.

At one point he found himself working in a pharmaceutical firm, doing research on diabetes. During the course of his work, Montignac discovered from the studies he reviewed that some 80% of diabetics were overweight. He found a report indicating that type ll (adult onset) diabetics who were put on certain types of carbohydrates succeeded in lowering their blood sugar and along with that, their weight went down. In some cases, their diabetes was brought completely under control. Convinced that he may have come across a true departure from what had been the conventional wisdom concerning diets, he decided to try eating the carbohydrates that were part of the diet protocol for the diabetic patients who were improving. He found that his weight started to drop steadily, and by the end of one year, he had lost over 30 pounds without reducing the amount of food that he ate. Montignac claims that this is because we don't gain weight because we eat too much, but because we eat the wrong food.

What will drive your commitment?

Dieting as we used to know it was a fickle enterprise. We either put our minds to following some fad of the moment that promised instant relief from obesity, or followed a nutritionist's careful plan that required counting and measuring food. Trying to remember the list of do's and don'ts didn't contribute to our comfort level, and soon we would find that we were either consumed with hunger, or dissatisfied with the choices of food that we were told to eat. Inevitably the diet would be abandoned. Failed again.

Failure leads to frustration that leads to desperation and hopelessness, until the prospect of making yet another effort to try to lose weight seems useless. And this may be the point that you've reached. Except that you're still overweight, and something must certainly be done to regain your health. The decision to try yet another method is the only way to go. Being overweight is not only a grooming blunder, it can lead to serious health problems. It is just a matter of time until the sinister side effects of obesity appear in the form of diabetes, high cholesterol, high blood pressure, and other related conditions.

The Biochemical Key method will allow you to get to where you want to go. You can even choose to lose weight faster or slower. The biochemical process has been studied sufficiently to tell you that if you are overweight, the problem is not that you're overeating - it's that you're eating the wrong food. The Biochemical Key method is fundamentally a matter of making correct food choices that will help you avoid cravings.

And so, once again, you're faced with the prospect of yet another diet! The difference now is that the Biochemical Key method follows a cause and effect process that you can adopt easily, and hunger will not get in the way of success this time. Understanding the rationale for food management that the Biochemical Key method advocates will help to motivate your resolve to keep it.

The paramount factors that make the remarkable results of the Biochemical Key possible and sustain permanent weight loss are features that defeat the weaknesses of diets, as follows:

1. With the Biochemical Key method, there is a distinct decline in hunger.

2. The Biochemical Key method is based on a theory that has been clinically tested. It is a hormonal approach to weight control. The Biochemical Key method advocates eating foods that actually lead to weight loss, and promotes balanced meals that permit eating till satisfied (without gorging).

3. Both #1 and #2 are related, and are facilitated by

eating foods that require a prolonged digestive process that will keep you satisfied, as you will learn.

4. Since the Biochemical Key method promotes a plan of balanced meals that are satisfying, your ideal weight can be maintained forever once it is reached. Counting and measuring food is not a convenient habit, and it is not part of the meal management program that you'll learn to follow.

The Biochemical Key teaches you how your metabolism is affected by the food you eat. It's a method that provides you with information about the biochemical process that has the potential to give you genuine control over your nutritional health.

The new nutrition is satisfying, curbs hunger, and eliminates cravings. It can improve digestion, correct constipation, lower blood pressure and cholesterol, and help control diabetes.

The Biochemical Key method:
* prevents feelings of food deprivation;
* prevents hunger between meals;
* obviates the need to count calories and measure food portions;
* prevents food cravings;
* stops rising irritability before meals;
* promotes mood stability;

* revives your energy level, cancels fatigue;
* improves skin tone.

To reach this state of well-being, you'll need the courage to change your eating habits. This is a difficult task for most people. We can try to cope with this issue in make-belief fashion, like this: Let's pretend that you were told that you had inherited a million dollars. Along with the gift, you were told that there's a magic formula for losing weight, but it's expensive. Of course you're interested. You're rich, you can afford it, and you want to enjoy your inheritance as a healthy person. How much of your inheritance would you be willing to give away to become thin? If your answer is not much, there's little chance that you'll apply what you will learn here, and there's not much reason to continue reading. But if you would be willing to spend a considerable amount, then you're motivated, and the right tool will help you achieve your goal - that tool is correct information to fuel your determination.

To follow the principles of the Biochemical Key, you will find yourself having to explain to friends and family who you are seated around the table with that you're managing your meals differently, and you won't eat certain foods. This instantly puts you in a class by yourself, which you may not find appealing, but it will be a worthwhile effort that will ultimately bring hope back again into your life.

You'll have the ability to make rational food choices

because the strong urge to succumb to unwelcome temptations will have abated with the decline of your hunger. And finally, the results that you'll start to see after the first three weeks will bring joy into your life. Seeing the puffiness melt away, feeling lighter, sleeping better, having more energy, and not having to cope with hunger between meals will motivate you to continue.

Please remember that in order to lose weight, you'll have to apply yourself. Using an analogy, let's consider this: if one wants to get from New York to Chicago, it can't be done by sitting in the living-room, at a restaurant, or in a phone booth. An appropriate vehicle must be found to do the job. Some vehicles are better than others. You have been using elevators. You've been going up and down (in weight), slimming and puffing! The Biochemical Key will give you control over how get to where you want to go, and you'll be able to control how fast or slow you will get there. The method is fundamentally a matter of making the right choices. It isn't a matter of eating less, unless you're gorging yourself at every meal. The message should be clear that to lose weight, you will have to do something!! Once again, you'll have to change your way of eating! But this time, you'll have the correct formula to get you going.

You should also know that managing your meals according to the Biochemical Key will help build your muscle mass. You'll see changes in your measurements before you see a change on the scale because muscle weighs more than fat, but takes up less room. This also explains the fact that with the Biochemical Key method, serious weight loss doesn't produce a haggard look!

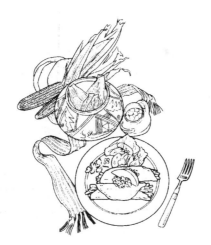

The key to the biochemical process

Some keys open doors, and some keys open the mind to new knowledge. The Biochemical Key explains the harmful effects of what has become one of the most popular food additives, one of the most favorite tastes, and one of the most unconsciously demanded food items that burdens our nutrition. That food item is sugar.

Sugar is a demon food.

Sugar contributes to hypertension and heart disease, raises cholesterol, and accelerates the symptoms of aging. It leads to fatigue, causes weight gain, dental cavities, and diabetes. Is there anything positive that can be said about sugar? No, simply because the glucose required for your brain and other tissues can be better derived from other, healthier foods such as brown rice, vegetables, fruits, etc.

Sugar is damaging. It is a slow-acting menace.

Americans consume about 62 kilos of sugar per person annually, which can partly be attributed to the popularity of their soft drink habit, which is a major industry in the U.S. Not many people know that a two-liter bottle of Coca-Cola contains approximately 45 cubes of sugar. A small can has about 14 cubes of sugar.

In the 1970s, Dr. Yudkin studied the damaging effects of sugar at a time when sugar was increasingly becoming a popular ingredient. Americans, he claimed, were becoming addicted to sugar and suffering poor health and obesity as a result. He reported that it was important to eliminate refined sugar from the diet. He claimed that if sugar were to be tested as a food additive, it would not be approved.

He wrote that the artificial sweetener cyclamate was ruled injurious to health after rats developed diseases because they were fed much higher amounts than a person would ordinarily consume. Rats fed smaller amounts of sugar, however, fared worse! They had enlarged and fatty livers, enlarged kidneys, and a reduced life span. He called this a concealed truth.

The fact is that humans have no known physiological need for plain sugar as an additive or in the form of a sweet. You don't have to eat a single teaspoon of white or brown sugar. In fact, eliminating sugar is the central key to a healthy diet.

Your first question should be - why?

Energy (sugar) from the food you eat can't stay in your blood stream. It must be used by your muscles and tissues. The remainder that is not used is stored as fat. The only way to control your weight is to control the amount of food you eat that raises your blood sugar level, because the insulin that is generated stores the unused sugar as fat. This is the essence of the hormonal approach to weight loss and weight gain, that is, weight control. It is this concept that lies at the root of correct meal management.

Simple! All that follows is clarification and elaboration!

Insulin is the primary hormone in the human metabolic system. The discovery of the influence of insulin is what opened the door to finally understanding the key to weight control.

Insulin plays a most critical part in the way the body uses carbohydrates and stores fat in the body. High levels of insulin in the bloodstream store fat and block the release of stored fat!

So now you can understand that low-calorie diets are ineffective when the foods they recommend cause the body to produce insulin. If you were told to eat dry rice cakes and baked potatoes on a low-calorie diet, you may be led to believe that you'll lose weight. But the truth is that you'll gain weight because white rice and potatoes turn to sugar in your blood, and the insulin that this releases will store the excess sugar as fat.

The restriction of sugar is necessary because it stimulates insulin secretion. The Biochemical Key method is based on the influence of insulin on metabolism. It also explains how eating protein leads to weight loss.

All foods are either carbohydrate, protein, or fat, and some contain all three.

Protein is derived from food that walked or swam or flew (except for soy and its derivatives), such as meat, cheese, fish, etc.;

While carbohydrates are derived from the ground where they grew, such as bread, potatoes etc.
(This ditty makes it easy to remember.)

Attention must be focused on carbohydrates because they turn to sugar in the body! It has been reported that currently the average American meal consists of some 90% carbohydrates. This alone can explain the prevalence of obesity that is raging in developed countries. With such a high consumption of carbohydrates, the high sugar content is causing insulin levels to keep soaring, and this contributes to the storage of fat, causing weight gain.

Now you can understand a puzzling situation. Most of us have been amazed to see photos of heavy men and women in the Soviet Union. What could possibly be the cause of their obesity when they had so little food to eat? They relied heavily on bread and potatoes. The high level of insulin that this diet generated caused the production of high levels of fat.

Don't blame yourself for having weak will power when you can't stop eating sweets, fresh bread, etc. It's now recognized that carbohydrates are as addictive to the overweight person as alcohol is to the alcoholic: the more cake, pasta, bread etc. one eats, the stronger the desire is to eat even more. This is because chronically high levels of insulin in the body also stimulate hunger. Most overweight people will admit that their hunger doesn't come from the belly. It's more properly described as a passion for particular foods, a feeling with unexplained origins.

Obesity is caused by an addiction. Seriously overweight people are preoccupied most hours of the day with thoughts about food - their every activity will provoke thoughts about food; taking a certain route to a destination will make them think about which stores they'll pass that have their "favorite" food; going to a family function produces thoughts about what food will be served. The uncontrollable craving is an abhorrent preoccupation that is wished away with every fiber, but can't be fought. Obesity destroys self-esteem and self-control. It's a physiological dependence. That is the definition of addiction.

It's not uncommon to hear someone say that they're dying for a piece of chocolate, or some other sweet. But how often have you heard someone say that they're dying to have a piece of cheese or a steak? Steak may be a favorite in some parts, but it's not usually referred to with the passion reserved for ice-cream.

Before the critical role of insulin was understood, this indeed was puzzling, because hunger can come very soon after a meal, when we should actually feel full. Or it can come on after starting to eat what was planned as a small snack but turned into a mini-feast, or from an uncontrollable temptation to eat that comes from just knowing there's cake in the kitchen. Now we know it as an addiction to carbs.

Follow the cool rule: **Never mix elements of different diets because you'll lose the benefits that are contained in each.** And, since the Biochemical Key is not a diet, but a lifetime of correct meal management, you mustn't, you won't have to, you shouldn't think about dieting!

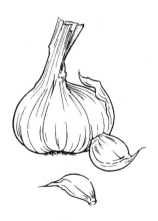

Insulin overload (hyperinsulinemia)

Now read carefully!

If you look in the mirror and you see an overweight, puffy person, you're looking at someone who is suffering from hyperinsulinemia. What is this terrible disease? It's not a disease at all, but a condition that develops after years of consuming foods that have a high sugar component.

How did that happen? The pancreas is the organ that generates the production of insulin. When carbohydrates are ingested, the starches turn to glucose (sugar), and the pancreas releases insulin in order to remove the excess glucose from the blood to transport it to the body's cells (liver and muscles). This provides us with our energy needs. In this manner, the sugar is removed from the blood, and the blood sugar level (or the glycemic level) is restored to normal.

However, after many years of eating too many foods that convert to too much glucose in the blood, the excess flow of insulin throws the metabolic system off balance. The insulin removes the glucose from the blood, but when there is too much glucose for the insulin to transport for use as energy, the insulin stores the rest of the glucose as fat. And that's how we gain weight - *too much sugar* generates *too much insulin*, which generates *the production of more fat.*

Just as serious is the trigger effect that chronically excessive insulin has. It encourages the kidneys to retain salt and fluid. This puts a heavier burden on the heart and raises blood pressure; it contributes to the stimulation of cholesterol production, which then thickens the muscular portion of the artery walls, increasing the risk of heart disease.

To simplify: The pancreas is the organ that generates insulin. When too much sugar has been entering the bloodstream for too long, the pancreas becomes over-worked. The clear and obvious damage done by an overstimulated pancreas is that it releases excess insulin, which signals the system to store the fat that is not needed for energy. This is the definitive circumstance that leads to obesity.

Training athletes are not affected in the same way as the ordinary person because their energy needs are much higher, which means that their bodies use the sugar that is in their blood for their energy output. Since their activity levels are high, there is no excess sugar that remains for the insulin to store as fat!! In fact, training athletes need carbohydrates to maintain their energy needs.

In the overweight person, the pancreas starts working as soon as food enters the system. This happens simply out of habit, even if the food contains no sugar. It is the over-production of insulin that causes the fat person to gain weight faster and easier than the thin person.

Hunger is the fat person's enemy. It is actually a craving

for carbohydrates that have been entering the body for so long. This can start soon after completing a three-course meal, or it can start with a snack that turns into a feast. Foods that cause the pancreas to generate excessive levels of insulin cause the blood glucose to drop to very low levels. This in turn stimulates the appetite and can cause the irritability we often feel when hungry. People who are overweight usually feel hungry due to the chronically high levels of insulin in their system.

Let's picture this process using a boat that is ferrying people from one shore to another many times every day. When the boat is new, and not many passengers are on board for each trip, it sails from one shore to the other where the passengers disembark, and a new group replaces them. If after many years the traffic becomes heavy and the captain increases the passenger load, too many passengers on each crossing will wear the boat down and cracks will begin to appear in the boat. To control the water that's seeping in through the cracks, the crew has to scoop the water out of the boat. When the crossings continue like this for too many years, with too many people on board, more water seeps into the boat, the cracks get bigger, and the crew is forced to work more furiously to get the water out. If the crew cannot do the job, additional crew will be hired.

In biological terms, the need for the extra crew is the onset of diabetes!

The extra crew that is taken on to keep the boat from

filling with water is the insulin that the pancreas is too "tired" to produce.

Why does the diabetic patient need more insulin when he is suffering from an overload of insulin? Because the diabetic person who has been eating too many carbohydrates for too long has an overburdened pancreas that can no longer manage to move the sugar out of the bloodstream into the cells. So more insulin is needed to do the job.

The pancreas is overworked because the cells that absorb the glucose have become insensitive over the years and won't allow the sugar in. This is caused by damage done to the receptors that coat the cells. They have been accessed for so long by so much insulin that they begin to resist, making the penetration of sugar into the cells too difficult.

The metabolic system deals with the unresponding receptor cells by accelerating pancreas activity to manufacture even more insulin to push the glucose into the cells. This surplus of insulin will promote the manufacture and storage of fat cells. And there you have it, you're gaining weight, and diabetes is just around the corner!

Prof. Walter willett collected data over a 10-year period. His conclusion was that there is a definite link between sugar and obesity. He was able to demonstrate that certain carbohydrates, eaten regularly, can lead to obesity, diabetes, and coronary disease. Willett's 1997 study at the Harvard School of Public Health showed that women who ate a low sugar, high-fiber diet had 2.5 times less risk of developing diabetes.

Sustained insulin overload creates a spiraling cycle: it is caused by a hunger, passion, addiction, and craving for carbohydrates, which provide the supply of sugar that triggers the secretion of more insulin. The heavier the person, the more sluggish he/she feels, the less exercise he/she does, and therefore, the less sugar is needed for energy, and so the insulin stores the sugar more efficiently as fat!

In the past, insulin overload was assumed to be a condition that seriously overweight people suffered from. It was not recognized that this condition was both a reaction to a high-sugar diet and also the cause of obesity. It could be that the difference between overweight people and people who are thin is that overweight people may have inherited a tendency for insensitive receptor cells. This would indicate that weight control is governed by the same metabolic system for both the fat and the thin. Fat people have receptor cells that resist, while in thin people the insulin can move the sugar into the cells easily. However, eating food that doesn't raise the blood sugar level will lead to the restoration of the cells' sensitivity, thus putting an end to insulin overload, and the fat will start to melt.

Essentially, the effect of carbohydrates on the body and the success of the Biochemical Key depends upon one's insulin sensitivity. Some people are naturally less carbohydrate sensitive than others, which requires their pancreas to secrete higher levels of insulin every time they eat. People whose cells are more sensitive and allow the insulin to do its job will tend to store less fat. So now it's easy to understand that two people who eat the same meal will be affected differently.

There is no medicine available for lowering insulin in the body. The only way to prevent insulin overload is through correct nutrition!

With the information that has become available about insulin overload, you can now lose weight and maintain an ideal weight level without the fear of sliding back. You can be in control. Diets that promote pills and potions are doomed because they cannot be maintained - and of course, they are expensive, not natural, and cannot contribute to optimal health in the long term. Eating correctly will reduce your bulging middle with surprising speed. That is, you will lose weight as well as inches. Your weight is regulated by what you eat, not how much you eat.

The Biochemical Key gives you maximum control, without compromising on the amount that you eat (unless you gorge yourself - and you know the difference)! The way to control your weight is to control your insulin levels. What you choose to eat will determine where this energy will go!

What about children? How is it that they can escape the damages of insulin?

Most children eat lots of high-sugar food with no serious consequences.

This is because in children, the cells are extremely sensitive to insulin, and so only small amounts are required to move the sugar out of the blood. With no excess insulin to store fat, they won't gain weight. Their cells are easily penetrated by the sugar that small amounts of insulin will transport from the blood. When they become adults, and their diets are too rich in carbohydrates, their receptor cells gradually lose their sensitivity to insulin. The result is insulin overload. This happens when the insulin levels are chronically excessive. After eating too much food that is high in carbohydrates, the blood sugar level rises over a long period of time and the cell receptors designed to respond to insulin begin to malfunction. The increase of obesity among children today is evidence of the popularity of fast foods that are loaded with carbs.

A note about fat: Fat doesn't increase insulin secretion. This means that fat can't be stored in the body without the help of carbohydrates. In fact, some hormonal diet researchers suggest eating only protein to lose weight. This, however, is not advisable. A diet based strictly on protein is a boring food plan. It can help you lose weight quickly, but it can't be sustained for a long time. And then, when you decide to drop the pure-protein diet, you'll find yourself very vulnerable to carbohydrates, and your weight will climb quickly. A diet of only protein is not a plan that will improve your health in the long term. But when you eat the right carbohydrates, much of the fat that's in the food you eat will pass right through your system without being stored.

There are different types of fat that we should be aware of. Saturated fats (animal fat) are undesirables because they cause an increase in cholesterol production. But monounsaturated, fats such as olive oil, are highly recommended because of their benefits. They help increase the HDL (the good cholesterol). The right kind of fat, like olive oil, avocados, almonds, macademia nuts and fish oils, can help lower insulin levels. Also, eating the right fat with a meal is beneficial because it helps give us the feeing of being full.

People who are overweight can't eat like ordinary people because they're in an insulin overload mode. But now you can do something about it! Lower your insulin level, and you may be sure that your body won't store fat. Not only will you not gain weight - your weight will come down.

Insulin overload also leads to high blood pressure, high cholesterol, and diabetes. So if you visit your doctor, and tests show that you're suffering from some or all of the above, you'll be put on medication indefinitely. This is the system that satisfies your doctor because your symptoms will decline; you become a patron of the pharmaceutical company that is selling you the medicine that keeps them in business; and you become the martyred party that is tied to medication that must be monitored regularly. What the medical professionals disregard and don't tell you is that

nutrients. It's easy to live with low-carb meals, and it's far better than a low-calorie diet that tells you to cut out fat, and eat less. The calorie-restricted diet keeps you hungry, and the next thing you know, you've stopped counting the calories. With the Biochemical Key method, hunger diminishes, giving you the ability to make the right food choices. There's no measuring and no counting.

All carbohydrates contribute to an increase of sugar in the blood. The body will break down carbohydrates into simple sugars (glucose, fructose or galactose) whether the carbohydrate is refined grains such as white rice or white bread or a more complex carbohydrate like starches or dextrins. The result will always be the same - conversion to glucose. The difference between them is that the carbohydrate in white bread is 100% available for conversion into glucose, while other sources of carbohydrate like fruits are perhaps only 50% available. Therefore, some carbohydrates have a higher "glycemic" effect than others.

The glycemic index: choosing the right carbohydrates

The glycemic index (G.I.) is a new way to look at carbohydrates in foods. Even though this system was developed over twenty years ago for diabetic patients, it is only now catching on with the general public.

Glycemia is the quantity of glucose that carbs cause the body to produce. The G.I. indicates the rate of absorption of glucose into the blood stream.

The G.I. is a numerical system that measures how fast and how much glucose was triggered in your blood by a carbohydrate - the higher the number, the greater the blood sugar response after eating.

Foods that have a high G.I. release glucose into the bloodstream quickly, and blood sugar levels soar shortly after eating them. So a low-G.I. food will cause a small, slow rise. Remember that high-G.I. food will trigger a dramatic insulin spike to deal with the sugar that enters the blood. The excess energy or calories will be stored as fat. By choosing higher G.I. foods, you're feeding your fat cells that will grow larger in size and multiply in number. The increase in body fat will slow your metabolism and take its toll on your energy level.

Eating too many high-G.I. carbohydrates for a long time will cause the system to generate high levels of insulin on a regular basis. Even if occasional meals are not heavy on carbs, the body responds out of habit, as though it is. The high insulin level also creates hunger, and the hunt for more carbs is on.

The lower the G.I. number, the slower the action, the less insulin is secreted, and less fat can be stored!

Carbs provide a quick sugar fix that may be recommended for athletes in training, but ordinary people can't burn the amount of energy that high-G.I. foods generate. Foods with a low glycemic index provide a steady small supply of glucose over several hours for the rest of us.

Before the glycemic index was created in the early 1980s, scientists assumed that simple sugars were absorbed and digested more quickly than complex carbohydrates. A lot of people still think that it is the foods that contain plain sugar that should be avoided. This distinction has finally been removed by the American Diabetes Association. Now it's known that simple sugars don't cause a blood sugar rise much more rapidly than some complex carbohydrates do, because these also convert to sugar in the body. The distinction that remains between simple and complex carbs is that simple carbs are sugars that contain no nutrition.

Many of the tested carbohydrates produced surprising results on the glycemic index (next section). The list shows that some complex carbohydrates, like baked potatoes, convert to a sugar level as high as simple sugar!

The way a food is prepared will affect the time it takes to break down in digestion. The glycemic index values take into account how easily a food is digested, the quantity of fiber it contains, the quantity of fructose (converts slowly), and the form in which the food is eaten. For instance, finely grated carrots are higher on the G.I. list than whole carrots: and cooking can make a starch more quickly digestible and so this raises its position on the glycemic index list. Cooked carrots have the highest G.I. value in the carrot family.

This is how the glycemic index (G.I.) list was created: researchers tested people who were given 50 gms of glucose. After a certain amount of time their blood was tested for insulin. The resulting insulin level was labeled

100 on the glycemic index, meaning that glucose equals 100 on the G.I. list. All other carbohydrates that were tested in the research were then ranked in relation to glucose. Some were the same as glucose, some were higher than 100, and some were lower. The lower a food is on the list, the more "weight friendly" it is.

The impact a food will have on blood sugar depends on many factors such as how ripe the fruit or vegetable is, how long it cooked, and the amount of fiber and fat the food contains.

It should be understood that not all lists are identical because researchers work differently. The numbers on different G.I. lists using glucose as a base value will be close but they won't all be identical. For instance, some fruits may have been riper in one study, or in another study a vegetable may have been cooked longer.

To manage your meals and snacks, you'll see that the essential differences between types of carbs are defined by their position on the G.I. The low-G.I. carbs will be the standard that you will choose from when you want to lose weight quickly and you don't want to cut down on the amount of food you eat.

Good carbs are low on the G.I. list, bad carbs are high on the G.I. list. Good carbs are vegetables that contain fiber, such as cabbage, broccoli, cauliflower, lettuce, green beans, leeks, asparagus and others. The fiber in low-G.I. carbs slows digestion and lowers the rate of insulin secretion. The amount of protein and the quality of fiber that are in carbohydrates also determine its glycemic index.

Eating low-G.I. carbs helps prevent drastic swings in blood glucose after meals and helps avoid high and low energy levels as well as appetite swings and mood fluctuations that occur throughout the day on a high carb diet.

When you stop eating high-G.I. foods and drinks, you rebalance the insulin stimulation in your metabolism. Dr. Andrew Weil of Harvard University - currently perhaps the most prominent writer and lecturer on integrative medicine - has come out strongly in favor of using the glycemic index as a guide to eating carbohydrates.

This is the logic that propels the Biochemical Key method of meal management. It would be absurd to ignore it: if insulin controls our metabolism, and the food we eat controls our insulin, then we can control our metabolism and maintain a high standard of health. This ability to control our metabolism, and therefore our weight, is the winning formula.

The wonder of protein

Understanding why you should be controlling the type of carbs you eat gives you the tool that completes only half the biochemical process. Although controlling your insulin production will help you avoid gaining weight, it's the protein in your diet that will actually help you lose weight. Protein helps promote weight loss.

Protein is found in two forms. Animal: fish, poultry, meat, eggs, and dairy products; and Vegetable: soy, almonds, hazelnuts, seeds, nuts, whole grains and certain legumes such as beans and lentils.

Since eating fat and protein won't add sugar to your bloodstream, they don't appear on the glycemic index. You're free to choose any protein that is low in fat, and eat to your satisfaction.

At this point you may be curious about why you have to continue to control the fat in your meals, if in fact you've been told that fat doesn't cause blood sugar to rise, and fat can't be stored without insulin. Why then should fat be avoided? It's true that fat won't be stored without the intervention of insulin, but this is true only when you eat a pure protein diet that has no carbs. As mentioned earlier, the Biochemical Key method doesn't encourage a pure protein diet. It recommends a *balanced* diet.

This means that along with the low-fat proteins that will

be part of every meal, only low-G.I. carbs should be on your menu when you want to lose weight fast. In time, you'll have small amounts of insulin released in your system, so you'll have to control the fat that you eat. The fat should be unsaturated fat such as olive oil and oils found in nuts and fish oil. These oils are important indeed, though in modest amounts, to maintain a higher HDL (the good cholesterol) level.

There are three benefits that are derived from eating protein, bearing in mind that it must be low-fat protein:

1. When you eat protein, the body can't receive its energy from an increase in sugar. This means that the system must use the fat that is stored in order to provide the energy that you expend. This is one of the ways that eating protein, actually helps you lose weight.

2. Because of its complex chemical composition, the protein uses more energy when it is being digested and broken down. The process of digesting a meal containing a large quantity of proteins elevates the metabolic rate to approximately 30% above average. The digestion of carbohydrates and fats usually raises the metabolic rate only about 4%. This means that the body uses more energy to digest proteins, and since the energy is taken from stored fat, this promotes weight loss.

3. Since the protein molecule is chemically complex,

digesting proteins also takes longer than digesting fat or carbs. This means that the feeling of satisfaction after a meal built around proteins can last for as long as three to eight hours. This has a definite effect on the time it will take until you begin to feel hungry. The longer the feeling of satisfaction is sustained, the lower and slower is the return of nagging hunger.

A balanced diet means eating protein at every meal along with certain carbs, of course, forever.

You can now understand that it's not the quantity of food that we eat, but the quality that is the major contributor to weight loss and weight gain. Eating food (low G.I. carbs) that won't lead to the storage of fat, and balancing that with food that will use your stored fat to get the energy you need (proteins), will effectively get your weight down. Stick to this way of managing your meals and you may eat as much as you need to feel satisfied, as long as you don't overeat (you know that feeling stuffed is uncomfortable, not satisfying).

Once you have begun managing your meals correctly, in a very short time, you'll notice that the cravings for 'just a little something' right after a meal, and between meals are beginning to subside. You'll stop thinking all the time (or almost all the time) about what you feel like snacking on. If you happen to catch sight of something appealing, the passion that used to force you to succumb to the temptation to eat won't have that same power over you, and you'll be able to weigh your decision more rationally. The Biochemical Key method helps curb your hunger, and that makes it easier to choose the right foods.

Eating low-fat protein encourages weight loss.
You should eat to feel satisfied.
Don't allow yourself to feel hungry.

A healthy, easy way to manage meals is something that you can live with for the rest of your life, and you'll do just that. We aren't talking about a diet that has a beginning and a final date. This is a way to manage meals that are healthy, balanced, and satisfying. The Biochemical Key offers a wide choice of foods that don't need any special effort to prepare, they're plentiful, easily accessible, and thoroughly nourishing. This conclusion is based on nutritional truths that tell us:

* Protein is an important food category.
* Unsaturated fats are necessary, but saturated fats are dangerous to the heart and blood vessels.
* High-fiber/low-starch carbohydrates contribute to your nutritional health.
* Insulin levels must be kept moderate and stable.

Conventional wisdom tells us that eating balanced meals, that is, all three food categories - carbohydrates, protein, and unsaturated fat - will give us the entire complement of nutritional needs that are necessary to maintain optimal health.

When you want to have a larger choice of carbs and you can cope with losing weight at a slower pace, you can choose from carbs that are higher on the G.I. list. Then, once you feel you look good, and you want to stay that way, you can add still more to your list of carbs to maintain your weight. But we're getting ahead of ourselves, because this is all clearly explained further on.

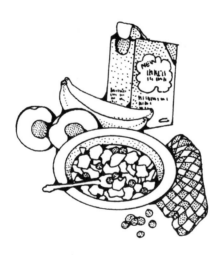

Bad, better, best:
The glycemic index list

Correct food choices for healthy living for a lifetime puts you in control of your health.

The glycemic index is a measure of the rate at which carbohydrates break down and release glucose into the bloodstream. Foods that have a high G.I. release glucose into the bloodstream quickly, and blood sugar levels climb shortly after eating them. Foods with a low G.I. provide a steady supply of glucose over several hours. Low-G.I. foods can be eaten without restriction.

The following is a list of the G.I. values that used glucose as the base value of 100. Some researchers use white bread as the base at 100, and then the numbers are higher for each item. You can check the Internet to add more items to this list compiled by R. Mendosa.

All the carbs on the list are ranked in relation to glucose.

The G.I. value of a food item is affected by how long it is cooked. The softer it becomes, the faster it is digested. You'll see from this list that carrots are in different positions, depending upon how they are prepared.

Each food category is ranked in order from low to high, so that you can readily see that the items at the top of a category convert more slowly to sugar in the body, and you'll choose from these to lose weight. You'll notice that some values even at the top of a category are too high to consider for your meals.

Legumes

Soy beans	18
Green lentils	23
Red lentils	30
Green beans	30
Dried beans	30
Black beans	30
Butter beans	31
Baby lima beans	32
Split peas	32
Chickpeas	33
Brown beans	38
Navy beans	38
Kidney beans	40
Pinto beans	42
Baked beans	43
Cooked broad beans	80

Breads

Pumpernickel	49
Rye, whole	50
Whole-wheat	55
Pita	60
Rye	64
Baguette	70
Bagel	72
White bread	72
Waffles	76
Hamburger roll	85

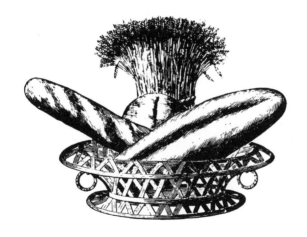

Cereals

All Bran	44
Whole-wheat sugar-free cereal	45
Oatmeal	53
Special K	54
Muesli	60
Cream of Wheat	66
NutriGrain	66
Oatmeal 1 min	66
Shredded Wheat	69
Refined unsweetened cereal	70
Cheerios	74
Puffed Wheat	74
Corn Bran	75
Rice Krispies	82
Cornflakes	83
Puffed Rice	90

Crackers

Wasa fiber rye	40
Rye	63
Kavli Norwegian	71
Saltine	72
Rice	85

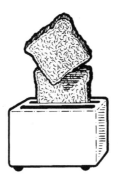

Vegetables

Raw carrots	30
Quinoa	35
Sweet potato	50
Boiled unpeeled potato	65
Beets	65
Boiled peeled potato	70
Pumpkin	75
Cooked carrots	85
Mashed potatoes	90
Baked potatoes	95
French fries	95
Potato chips	95

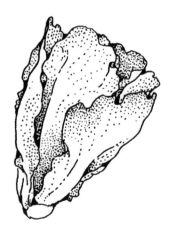

Fruit

Cherries	22
Plums	24
Grapefruit	25
Apricot	30
Banana, unripe	30
Strawberries	32
Figs	35
Dried apricots	35
Pear	36
Apple	38
Grapes	43
Orange	43
Kkiwi	52
Fruit cocktail	55
Raisins	55
Mango	55
Cantelope	60
Banana	62
Apricot, canned	64
Raisins	64
Pineapple	66
Watermelon	72

Grains

Pearl barley	22
Rye	34
Chickpeas	36
Wheat, whole	41
Bulger	47
Rice, parboiled	47
Buckwheat	54
Basmati rice	55
Brown rice	59
Long grain rice	60
Cornmeal	68
Sweet corn	70
Millet	75
Popcorn	85
White rice	88
Rice, instant	91

Dairy products

Milk	34
Chocolate milk unsweetened	34
Yogurt	38
Ice cream (vanilla)	50
Maltose beer	110

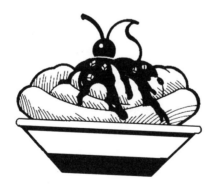

Pasta

Soy vermicelli	30
Vermicelli	35
Spaghetti, al dente	40
Whole-grain pasta	40
Macaroni	46
Durum Linguine	50
Whole-wheat pasta	50
Well-cooked spaghetti	55
Ravioli	70

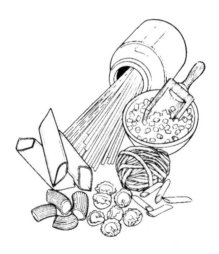

Other

Soy nuts	20
Peanuts	20
Sugar-free jam	22
Fructose	22
Chocolate with at least 70% cocoa	22
Chocolate bar	70
Honey	85

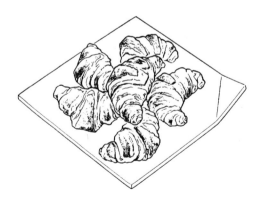

"Free" vegetables

This is a list of vegetables that are free, which means you can eat these without limit. They can be sauteed, boiled, roasted, grilled, baked, stewed, etc. They are 15 or lower on the G.I. list.

Green vegetables
Tomatoes
Eggplant
Zucchini
Garlic
Onions
Lettuce
Mushrooms
Celery
String beans
Green peppers
Scallions
Broccoli
Asparagus
Cabbage
Cauliflower
Brussel sprouts
Cucumber
Radish

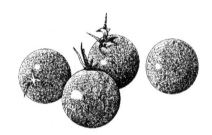

Your eating strategy: the impact

Everyone develops their own eating habits according to a unique set of needs. What you've discovered by now, however, is that without exception, we're all vulnerable to the ravages of soaring insulin levels. The individual differences between us are in the extent to which our receptor cells have become desensitized, and don't readily accept the glucose to be absorbed (or scooped - like the sailing crew trying to keep the boat afloat) into our cells. A complex scientific analysis is not necessary to calculate who falls into the least sensitive category. The mirror tells the truth. The more overweight we are, the more insulin our pancreas is secreting, and the longer it will take to tame our metabolism. It takes a bit of time to reach an ideal weight, but on the Biochemical Key method, results start to become apparent quickly - many people say they feel a difference after two weeks.

Doesn't it sound logical? Doesn't it make sense? Doesn't it sound easy?

You must have come to that conclusion at the beginning of the book.

Now let's get practical.

The first hurdle is to decide that you're going to reclaim your good health and fine appearance. You understand the theory - even though you'll probably want to reread this several times to get the information clearly stored in your mind.

So it's settled. You're going to follow the Biochemical Key method for your meal management, and this means that you've set your mind to do what it takes to succeed. Your previous resolutions sounded identical, right?

Maybe, but this time there's a difference. You now know that operatively, the weak link that spoiled your worthy plans to lose weight in the past is actually the strong component (not the only one) of the Biochemical Key, because now you'll be able to control your hunger, and your body won't resist the weight loss as it did on low-calorie diets. You also know that whenever you like you can reach out for a low fat protein, and you can eat till you feel satisfied (not stuffed).

This is a lifetime strategy of meal management because our biochemical system doesn't change. A menu of potatoes, white flour, white rice, corn, sweets, and other high G.I. foods will always cause the same reactions that will put us in a weight-gain mode.

Years of eating high G.I. food regulated your pancreas to release high levels of insulin. Even when you had a meal that was relatively low in starch and sugar, your system reacted habitually and released more insulin than was necessary. This will explain why during short intervals when you knew you were eating very little, you were still gaining weight, or at the very least, you weren't losing weight. As your new pattern of eating begins to cause a slower, lower release of insulin, your metabolism will begin to change. This takes time, and it is different for each person. The more attempts you have made in the past to lose weight, the longer it will take for you to become accustomed to this new system that operates consistently to restrict the production of insulin.

With the reduction of insulin, you will begin to feel satisfied, and stay satisfied for hours. Your weight will start to drop quite early on - probably by the end of the third week you'll start to see results. But you will reach a plateau approaching the sixth week, perhaps, and you will begin to doubt the merits of your efforts. Keep with it. You'll outsmart your metabolism. It's likely that by the end of 12 weeks, your insulin production will have begun to respond to your new food intake, rather than secrete by habit, and you'll notice that your fat deposits are beginning to melt. This becomes more clearly obvious in men whose weight is centered in their middle. You'll begin to sense that the cravings you had are weaker, and that the temptation to eat is beginning to decline. You also won't feel bloated after a three-course meal.

You should be aware that weighing in every day is a frustrating experience. First of all, you can weigh yourself every day, but your weight should be calculated by the weekly average. At the beginning, depending on the quantity of proteins that you have been accustomed to eating and the corresponding density of your muscle mass, you may find that the scale is not responding. You aren't losing weight. This is because protein contributes to an increase of muscle mass while reducing the fat deposits. Since muscle weighs more than fat, but takes less room, you may weigh the same, but you'll see that your measurements are changing. This is why it's important to weigh yourself and measure your chest, waist and hips before you start on the fast track. The realignment of your form will very soon include weight reduction. It must happen - you're intervening in a biochemical process, and you'll see the results on the scale, too.

You may find at the beginning that you'll be constipated. You may become light-headed. You're reacting to the insulin changes. All these symptoms and more - remember Ada's letter - will disappear in a short time. (Consult your doctor before you start, to rule out health problems.) Soon you'll begin to feel more energetic, more in control of your moods. You'll feel an improvement in your sleep, your digestion, your appearance, and more.

What to do: the fast track

Don't read this section until you've read everything that came before it. Unless the theory is understood, this section will not be meaningful

The Biochemical Key offers three tracks for meal management. The fast track is for everyone. This track, although broad enough in terms of the choice of foods, is more restrictive than the other tracks, but it is also the most vigorously effective. It is on this track that you will see the fastest results. It is recommended that everyone start the Biochemical Key meal management on the fast track.

1. Plan every meal around protein. Your choice of protein should come from meat, fish, soy meat, tofu or poultry, rather than from a food that merely contains a small portion of protein, like a legume. Make certain that it is a low-fat meat protein, or a high-fat fish protein such as salmon, mackerel etc. At the beginning, you will be surprised to discover that until now, you have been eating more carbs than you had thought. This is a major change as you start on your low-fat protein, high-fiber/low-G.I. carb plan.

2. Along with low-fat protein, choose vegetables that are *up to 15 on the G.I.* They can be broiled, lightly fried, sauteed, steamed or raw.

3. Try to restrict your fruit intake for the first six weeks. Low-G.I. fruits are fine on the other tracks because their sweetness is derived from fructose, which is digested more slowly than sugar.

4. It is recommended not to drink fruit juices on this track. They contain no pulp, and therefore no fiber, so they're digested quickly.

5. You may choose from a wide range of low-fat dairy products, but do not consider cheese as your main portion of protein. You need more protein per meal than is contained in cheese. If your cholesterol is high, don't eat hard cheeses that ordinarily have a higher fat content.

6. We can all benefit from eating only the whites of eggs. The yolks are not recommended when cholesterol is a factor. Yolklessness is hardly noticed in an omelette or a fried egg, and you can make up the volume by adding more whites. Having four eggwhites at a meal is not bizarre if you like eggs.

7. Use extra virgin olive oil. You may use canola occasionally, or even sunflower oil. But never never use margarine because of the hydrogenated oil that it contains.

8. Drink about eight glasses of water every day. Water is necessary to keep your system fit when your body is burning stored fat. You will in any case feel more thirsty. You can increase the water you drink by having a glass in the morning when you wake up. Then, after every meal freshen your mouth with a glass of water. You'll be thirsty between meals, so carry water with you and by the end of the day you'll find that you have consumed eight glasses or more.

9. You may want to continue drinking diet soda, but you'd be far better off drinking water. Doing this will wean you off the sweet taste that has become so much a part of your diet.

10. It is advisable for your coffee to be decaffeinated. One researcher found that regular coffee causes a rise in insulin.

11. Don't allow yourself to be hungry. Eat at least three meals a day - remember that eating low-fat protein promotes weight loss, so have a snack when you feel the need.

12. Snack on protein (low-fat cheese strings, low fat sliced chicken,etc.). You'll find it more satisfying than a raw carrot or sliced cucumber, though these are fine if they tempt you.

13. We all have food preferences that may cause us to eat more of one type of food consistently at the expense of another. To maintain balanced nutrition most medical professionals recommend taking a multi-vitamin daily.

14. The benefits of Omega-3 fatty acids are praised by most medical professionals. Found in fish oil, its components have a positive effect on the brain and the heart, and they are reputed to work to alleviate chronic diseases. They also control insulin production. Eat fatty fish several times a week, and take a fish oil capsule every day.

15. Yes! Have one glass of dry red wine with your dinner (or lunch). Don't drink it alone without food.

The fast track will help rebalance your metabolism by normalizing your pancreas so that it can relax the release of insulin. At the beginning you'll find it an effort to change your eating habits. You'll find:

* You're shopping differently. Look for proteins that you never ate before, check out new food stores to find different products, make sure you have a supply of protein on hand in your kitchen, at work, even in your car - keep dry nuts handy.

* You want to be clear about the choices of food that you'll be making from among the G.I. carbs that are not higher than 15 while you are on the fast track. Your meals

on this track should consist of protein and vegetables. Keep them varied so that you feel satisfied.

* You will think about food in a different way. You won't be able to rely on a quick sandwich, or the ordinary processed snacks. Start to think about which store has the better sliced meat, where you can pick up good herring, smoked salmon, and soy snacks.

* Vegetarians can get their required portions of protein from eating soy derivatives such as tofu that are available in different forms (the processed products are not recommended, unless the ingredients say otherwise).

* We can all benefit from eating soy foods. Soybean derivatives are an excellent source of protein. It is among the lowest food on the glycemic chart. In addition, it is the only bean that contains more protein than carb. Also, soybeans are loaded with fiber, including the soluble type that slows down rising blood sugar. Soybeans are said to improve thyroid function. This can help keep metabolism high, which will promote weight loss. There are many other benefits from soy products that you can read about elsewhere. (Soy sauce and soybean oil, however, contain very little soybean protein.)

* Approach eating in restaurants differently. Read through the menu and ask for a description of the items that appeal to you. Be assertive. Have the courage to ask for changes in a dish, so that it doesn't contain foods that are above 15 on the G.I., and it becomes a good choice for you.

* The best bread to eat is whole-grain rye, in terms of the glycemic results. If it doesn't please your taste buds, try whole-grain wheat bread.

All of the above are new to you as you start to manage your meals correctly. But in time, it will become as much a part of you as the damaging foods are that you're eating now. Change is more difficult for some people than others. It's not a matter of eating different foods, it's the struggle with change that some find disturbing. So, to follow this logic, it may be safe to say that if you have difficulty with change, once your meal management is correct, you'll have a hard time changing back to your old damaging meals. For instance, can you think of eating sugar again without the knowledge that you now have?

Embarking on a path that has not yet been traveled into unknown territory is intimidating, and the route is crowded with unforeseen obstacles that will raise questions. Your perceptions of the Biological Key method are likely to be different from others'. Chances are you'll have stored information that is different from what someone else would have absorbed. So, before you start, read this with someone who has also decided to do something about their health. *Team up with them.* You can be there for each other to answer questions, share doubts and exchange suggestions. The support that you will share can help make this journey an enjoyable one.

You will want to stay on the fast track till you've

reached your ideal weight - which can be what you decide that it should be according to how you look and how you feel. You can stay on the fast track as long as you like without the worry of going to an extreme because basically you'll be eating balanced meals. Your nutritional needs will be met (unless you're suffering from a condition that will put you in a category of special needs. You'll learn this from the visit to your doctor, as recommended earlier).

Nothing has been said about exercise, because we're dealing with meal management. But since the aim of good meal management is good health, and this can be achieved by keeping in good shape, then it's an issue to consider. Too many of us don't have the opportunity to challenge our bodies to reach a state of healthy physical fatigue. A small effort will go a long way. I'll tell you how I created a routine that works for me:

* Every morning I start the day with a glass of water.

* I drink my second glass while working out in front of the TV.

I taped a load of easy exercise programs that I do every day at a time that is convenient for me. When I started, I could barely get into the second exercise. Now, I can finish every program. So if the only thing you can do is lift your arms and legs slightly, do it. Let the rythmn of the music stir you. Follow the simplest exercises to the best of your ability. Soon you'll be very proud of how far you've come.

* My third glass is used to down the multi-vitamin and fish-oil capsule.

* I don't eat until about one hour later - this helps the system dip into stored fat for energy.

* Now I'm ready to meet the day feeling energized physically, and emotionally comfortable, knowing that I'm being good to myself again today!

This routine is now a matter of habit - a good habit that needs no deliberation and no planning. Everyone deserves pampering, and this is one way of getting it, if only you can recognize that it's a good way to get it!

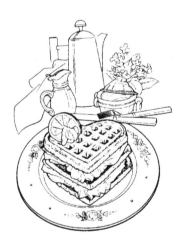

The main track

On the main track, you can add the G.I. carbs that are *up to the high 30s on the list.* You can have lentils, quinoa, whole-wheat couscous, al dente spaghetti, chickpeas, peanuts and almonds. But these should be eaten in limited quantities. You can have as much as you like of low G.I. vegetables and low-fat protein (without gorging). You'll continue to lose weight on carbs that are in the 30s, but at a slower pace. This track is less restricting in terms of the variety of choices.

Continue to build your meals around protein, and drink plenty of water. All your meals should be balanced, with low-fat protein and low G.I. carbs.

Add fruit up to 35 on the G.I. list. Whole fruit is better than fruit juice which doesn't have the pulp, so the fiber is removed.

For chocoholics and those who have heard about reports that chocolate acts as an antioxidant, which is beneficial, you can snack on bits of chocolate, providing it's the kind that has at least 70% cacao, which is available in most large supermarkets. It's not baking chocolate that no one would want to eat, but fine, delicious bitter chocolate. The proportion of cacao content is usually placed prominently on the package.

Your weight will go down steadily but more slowly on

this track. With your hunger harnessed, you'll find that your old weaknesses for high G.I. carb foods have become less compelling, and as time goes by, they will be easier to resist.

By now you'll be feeling good about yourself, your appearance, and your energy level.

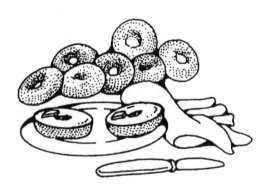

Forever

On this track, you can eat up to the 50s on the G.I. list. The choice on this track is the widest, and you won't gain weight, or lose weight. This track will be your regular guide to sustaining the weight that you want to stay at.

If your physical energy output level does not change, meals that are built around courses that are higher than the mid-50s on the G.I., will increase your insulin production and contribute to the storage of fat, and soon you'll be back on the path to gaining weight again.

It should be understood that you can eat food up in the 30s on the G.I. without worry about the amount you eat. But *carbs that are above this G.I. level should be eaten in limited portions.*

Eating wisely forever will mean that this method of meal management will never change - low-fat protein and low-G.I. carbs will dominate every meal. You will always be able to control your nutritional health because you now have the knowledge of how the biochemical process functions in the body, and since knowledge is power, you can use this information to give you the ability to control your weight.

Dealing with "relapses" is not complicated, and this will arise from time to time. At most parties, you'll be wise to start filling up on friendly foods (till the 30s). You may find that although the food is appealing, and there is enough to choose from among the meat, fish and vegetable fancies on offer, you decided here and there to taste things you haven't had in a long time, and soon you find you've eaten a whole serving of bad carbohydrates. Don't panic. You won't be knocked too far off base. The simple solution is to have only protein for the first two meals the next day. That should help to put you back on track.

What is likely to help put an end to sinning is that after eating high G.I. carbs, you'll most likely feel the effects physically - eating junk will probably cause belching, gas, and general gastric discomfort.

Be biochemically wise and aware of the pitfalls - friends that tempt you, appealing aromas, passing open bakeries, thoughts that you deserve a food reward, stresses that are not resolvable immediately, etc. You'll be your own best friend if you always make sure to have access to protein choices, for example, on the way home from work you know that the store across the street has great low-fat hard cheese. It will keep you going until you get home for dinner, etc., so have some.

This is a lifetime commitment that will give you healthy, well-balanced, nutritious, and satisfying meals. You'll regain the once-fit person who is still inside of you. The onset of the disabling symptoms of old age will be delayed for many, many years, and you'll have the luxury of enjoying a fine quality of life after retiring. We haven't been educated to look forward to old age, but with good health to accompany us there, it becomes a wonderful prospect. All that free time, and all that new energy to enable us to enjoy it!

So, go get healthy!

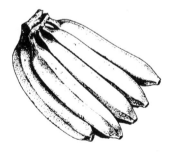

Your good food guide for the fast and medium tracks

Breakfast Options

Egg whites scrambled, boiled, fried, poached

Chopped egg whites with a spoon of crushed chickpeas and a dash of mayonnaise

Whole-grain french toast

Mushroom omelette

Herring

Smoked salmon

Low-fat cream cheese

Low-fat cottage cheese

Lacurda fish

Mackerel

Sardines with tomatoes and onions

Open lettuce and tomato sandwich with mustard on whole-grain bread

Plain yogurt with chopped cucumbers and tomatoes, salt & pepper

No-fat sour cream with strawberries, blackberries or blueberries

Unsweetened granola (some have no sugar, but beware of maltose, etc.)

Whole-grain rye bread
Genuine pumpernickel bread
Wasa fiber rye crackers
Decaf coffee
Tea, skim milk
No potatoes
No white rice
No corn
No sugar
No food made with white flour
No more than two thin slices of whole-grain bread per day

Lunch and dinner options

Fish & Meats
Tuna
Herring
Liver paté
Dry sausage
Lean cold cuts
Chicken/turkey without skin
Lean hamburger
Lean steak
Smoked, marinated, baked, broiled salmon
 Sardines, mackerel, cod, trout, haddock, etc.

Others
Goat cheese
Low-fat hard cheeses
Eggs
Fish soup
Mozzarella
Tofu
Soy
Low-fat cottage cheese
Burger meat substitute

Vegetables
(raw, quickly steamed, or lightly sautéd)

Asparagus
Tomatoes ✓
Cucumbers ✓
Peppers
Celery ✓
Mushrooms .
Green beans .
Leeks
Cabbage
Cauliflower ✓
Spinach ✓
Lettuce ✓
Broccoli

Raw carrots ✓
Artichokes
Avocado

Learn to read the ingredients on a package before buying!

Snacks for the Fast Track

A snack is not a meal, and the amounts consumed should be just enough to give you a lift, relieve your hunger, and leave you with a good taste in your mouth.

Soy nuts, peanuts, almonds, sliced low-fat cheeses, cottage cheese, sliced meats, etc. are good, and these can be added to raw low G.I. vegetables.

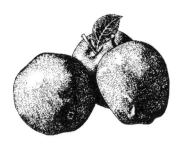

Yummie recipes
that work for you

For your convenience, here are easy to prepare, biochemically friendly recipes that are delicious.

Unusually healthy

As-Much-As-You-Like Salad Dressing

Ingredients:
1 cup plain yogurt
1 level teaspoon regular mustard
1 level teaspoon garlic powder
salt & pepper to taste

Preparation:
Mix the dry ingredients in a small bowl.
Add to a cup of yogurt.
Mix vigorously.
Pour over salad, fish, spaghetti, noodles, or anything dry that is enhanced by a light sauce.

Divine

Heavenly hamburgers

Ingredients:
1 cup dry ground soy bits (these have the texture of ground chicken when soaked and cooked)
1 teaspoon onion powder
1 level teaspoon hickory powder or liquid smoke
1 teaspoon garlic powder
2 teaspoons fructose crystals or powder
salt & pepper to taste
1 kilo lean ground beef

Preparation:
In a bowl, soak soy bits in water for 10 minutes.
Pour out the liquid.
To the wet soy bits add all the ingredients except the meat.
Mix well.
Add the meat to the mixture.
Knead the meat and soy mixture well for several minutes till all the ingredients are well integrated.
Divide the mixture into 7 or 8 balls (depending on the size of your portion preference for each hamburger).
Flatten the balls on a hard surface so that the middle of

each burger is thinner than the edges (to allow faster and more thorough cooking).

Heat olive oil in a large frypan and fry.

Eat as much as you like!

Scrumptious

The Joy of Soy Spaghetti Sauce
(tastes like spaghetti sauce with ground chicken)

Ingredients:
1 large onion, chopped
4 cloves fresh garlic, crushed
olive oil
1 cup canned tomato paste
2 cups crushed canned tomatoes
1 cup dry soy bits
1 level teaspoon oregano
1/3 cup dry red wine
3 drops of liquid artificial sweetener
salt & pepper to taste

Preparation:
Drain the soaked soy bits.
In a medium size pot, fry the onion and garlic in olive oil.
When transparent, add the drained soy bits.
Add the remaining ingredients.
Bring to a boil. Cook covered for 15 minutes on the lowest flame, stirring occasionally

The best ever

Oven Roasted Vegetable Chunks

Ingredients:
1 eggplant
4 courgettes
2 medium sweet potatoes
1 onion
1 red pepper
1 green pepper
1 cauliflower
olive oil
hyssop
2 teaspoons garlic powder
1 teaspoon sweet paprika
salt & pepper to taste

Preparation:
It is not necessary to peel the vegetables. Just wash and trim.
Grease a large oven roasting pan with olive oil.
Cut each vegetable in chunks.
Place the vegetable chunks on the greased pan, spread out as much as possible.
Sprinkle with the spices.
Drip olive oil on the vegetables.

Place in a 200C oven.

After 1/2 hour, the juices will begin to run.

Using a wide wooden spoon, mix the vegetables to get even exposure to the heat .

Bake another 30 minutes.

Remove from the oven immediately.

Unexpectedly exciting

Sautéd Chinese Tofu

Ingredients;
Freeze 660 grams (1 1/2 lbs) of firm tofu (this will give it a more solid texture)
5 cloves garlic
5 green onions
4 celery stalks
1 green pepper
1 egg
salt and pepper
(whole-wheat flour, optional)
1/2 teaspoon sweet paprika
1 teaspoon garlic powder
2 tablespoons soy sauce
1 level teaspoon ginger
1/4 to 1/3 cup water
olive oil

Preparation:
Defrost the tofu overnight.
Dice the green onion, garlic, pepper, and celery small pieces and leave in a bowl.
Break an egg into a clean bowl.
Add 2 teaspoons paprika; salt and pepper to taste.

Squeeze the liquid out of the block of tofu.

Slice the block into small triangles by cutting strips, and then cutting the block across to the right / left

Separate the pieces and add to the egg and mix well until all the tofu is covered with the egg mixture.

Put enough olive oil into a pan to sauté the tofu for 5 minutes, mixing.

Empty into a bowl.

Add more olive oil to the pan and heat.

Sauté the diced vegetables for about 3 minutes. Then add the tofu. When the mixture is consistent, add the soy sauce, ginger and water. Let cook for about 1/2 minute.

Eat as much as you like!

Tantalizing treat

Nice 'n' Easy Sesame Tofu

Ingredients:
1 egg
660 gms (1 1/2 lbs) tofu
2/3 cup sesame seeds
cumin
ginger
salt and pepper
2 teaspoons paprika
olive oil

Preparation:
Defrost the tofu the evening before.
Beat the egg.
Add the cumin and ginger (to taste) to the egg.
Add the paprika.
Mix well.
Squeeze the block of tofu to remove the water, and slice.
Mix the tofu into the egg mixture, and mix well.
Pour the sesame into a bag.
Add the tofu to the bag and mix well.
Grease a baking pan with olive oil.
Place the prepared tofu in the pan.

Bake in a 200C oven for about 20 minutes, turning after 7 minutes.

When it looks ready, remove from oven.

Eat as much as you like!

Heavenly, filling, and healthy!

Cholent Cheat (because in a modest quantity it does no harm to the biochemical process)

Ingredients:
1 cup dry soy bits, soaked and drained
2 medium / large onions, chopped
3 cloves garlic, crushed
1 cup red beans
2 sweet potatoes cut in large chunks
2/3 cups whole-wheat grains and/or pearl barley
salt and pepper to taste
2 drops liquid artificial sweetener
1 tablespoon red wine vinegar
1 can crushed tomatoes
olive oil

Preparation:
Soak beans overnight.
Cover the bottom of a large pot with olive oil and heat.
Sauté onions and garlic.
Add remaining ingredients.
Add just enough water to barely cover.
Cover and bring to a boil (don't mix after boiling).
Leave in a slow cooker or on a hot-plate overnight.

Enjoy as a side dish.

Simply scrumptious

Simple chicken or turkey shnitzel

Ingredients:
6 slices of schnitzel, pounded flat
2/3 cup plain oat bran (you have to stock up on healthy ingredients, remember?)
2 heaped teaspoons sweet paprika
1 heaped teaspoon garlic powder
salt and pepper to taste
olive oil

Preparation:
Wash the schnitzel slices.
Pour all remaining dry ingredients into in a plastic bag.
Hold the bag closed and shake vigorously.
Place the schnitzels into the bag and shake till they are completely covered with mixture.
Grease a baking pan generously with olive oil.
Place schnitzels in the pan and turn to oil them on both sides.
Oven-fry in a hot oven for 15 minutes if very flat, or 20 minutes if rather thick.
Remove immediately when ready.

Eat as much as you like!

Deliciously strange

Quinoa with fried onions
(not a grain, not a legume - it's in the fruit family)

Ingredients:
1 cup quinoa
1 large onion, finely diced
salt & pepper to taste
1 teaspoon onion powder
olive oil
1 teaspoon wine vinegar

Preparation:
Sauté onions in hot olive oil and remove to a bowl.
Wash quinoa and drain.
Add to the sautéing onions to dry.
Add boiling water (2 cups water per 1 cup quinoa) to the quinoa.
Cook, covered, on lowest flame for close to 15 minutes.
When soft but still grainy, turn heat off and leave uncovered (water should be almost totally absorbed).
Immediately add onion powder and wine vinegar and blend.

Eat as much as you like!

Veritably Middle Eastern

Shakshuka

Ingredients:
1 1/2 kilo ripe tomatoes
1 can crushed tomatoes
2 onions
2 red peppers
3 garlic cloves
olive oil
eggs
salt and pepper to taste
cumin to taste
1 cup dry ground soy bits

Preparation:
Cut tomatoes into cubes.
Dice onions and garlic.
Dice red peppers.
Sauté onions and garlic.
Add red peppers, mix and sauté.
Add tomatoes and spices to taste.
Add crushed tomatoes.
Cook covered on a low flame for 10 minutes.
Drop dry soy bits into the mixture slowly to thicken, and mix.
Break the eggs on mixture in pan.
Cook covered another 10 minutes.

Eat as much as you like!

Casserole king

Vegetable casserole

Ingredients:
2 sweet potatoes
2 onions
3 cloves garlic
2 green peppers
4 green onions
1 small cauliflower
2 courgettes
3 eggs
1/2 cup oat bran
salt and pepper to taste
olive oil
1/2 teaspoon cumin
teaspoon hyssop (za'atar)
1 teaspoon soup powder (your preference)
1/2 cup dry soy bits

Preparation:
Dice the vegetables.
Sauté the onions and garlic in olive oil.
Add all the remaining ingredients.
Grease a baking pan, and preheat it in a medium oven.
Pour mixture into the hot pan.
Bake in a medium oven for about 1 hour (until the top is brown and crusty).

Eat as much as you like!

Schnitzel with a difference

Soy-Coated Schnitzel

Ingredients:
1/2 cup dry ground soy bits
6 slices flat turkey or chicken schnitzel
olive oil
2 teaspoons sweet paprika
salt and pepper to taste
1/2 teaspoon madras curry powder
splash of soy or whole-wheat flour

Preparation:
Place the soy bits in a plastic bag.
Add all dry ingredients except schnitzel.
Shake well.
Add schnitzel and shake.
Grease a Teflon pan well and heat.
Fry schnitzel on both sides till ready.

Eat as much as you like!

A royal meal

Baked turkey breast

Ingredients:
a whole turkey breast
salt and pepper to taste
1 teaspoon Worcester sauce
1 teaspoon balsamic vinegar
2 teaspoons paprika
1 teaspoon olive oil
1/2 teaspoon powdered ginger
1 teaspoon fresh or powdered garlic
Add to the pan as an option: 2 or 3 sweet potatoes, broccoli (and other vegetables you like)

Preparation:
Wash turkey breast and place it in a broad roasting pan.
Place cut sweet potatoes around the turkey.
In a bowl, mix all ingredients (can be thickened by adding unrefined flour if desired).
Spread over the turkey.
Bake, covered, in a 200C oven for 70 to 90 minutes (depending upon your preference).
Remove from oven immediately.

Eat as much as you like!

Meat treat

Baked tomato meat loaf

Ingredients:
1 kilo minced lean beef
1 cup dry soy bits
1 chopped onion
3 cloves minced garlic
1 can crushed tomatoes
1/4 cup balsamic vinegar
salt and pepper to taste
oregano

Preparation:
Soak the soy bits, drain them, and place in a bowl.
Add onions, garlic, salt and pepper and mix well.
Add minced meat to the bowl.
Knead the meat mixture well.
Put into a loaf or round roasting pan.
Pour the crushed tomatoes into the empty bowl.
Add the remaining ingredients and mix well.
Pour the tomato mixture over the meat.
Bake in a 175C oven for 1 hour.

Eat as much as you like!

Fish favorite

Baked salmon

Ingredients:
a small to medium-sized side of salmon filet
lemon juice from 1/2 lemon
1/4 cup soy sauce
pepper to taste
1/2 teaspoon ginger
lots of crushed garlic
1 teaspoon paprika
olive oil

Preparation:
Wash and place fish on a pan greased with olive oil.
Mix the remaining ingredients in a bowl.
Pour over fish.
Cover the pan.
Place in a 175C oven, covered, and bake for 1/2 hour
(more, if the filet is thick). When the center is light pink
and flaky, the fish is ready.
Remove from oven as soon as it is ready.

Eat as much as you like!

What health tastes like!

Guacomole

Ingredients:
2 avocados
1 large tomato
3 medium-sized garlic cloves
1 medium onion
2 tablespoons olive oil
salt and pepper to taste
2 teaspoons lemon juice

Preparation:
Cut tomato in tiny pieces and put in a bowl.
Peel the avocado and add to bowl.
Finely chop the onion and garlic and add.
Add remaining ingredients.
Cut into the mixture with a chopper until it is in fine bits, not a cream.
Eat with whole-wheat bread or crackers.

Have as a side dish.

Eat-to-lose-weight

All-you-can-eat veggie soup

In a large pot or pressure cooker, place:
3 stalks of diced celery
1 diced green pepper
5 green onions
1 medium head of sliced cabbage
1 cup dry soy bits, soaked
1 can crushed tomatoes
3 liters water

Add salt, pepper, 1/2 cup red wine, 1 teaspoon cumin.

Add water to cover, and cook until the vegetables are tender.

(If you have no patience for fingerwork, slice only the cabbage, and cut the rest of the vegetables in half to cook. When ready, use a hand processor to chop all the vegetables in the pot as finely as you like - 5 seconds should do it!)

Eat as much as you like!

Mock Cheese Balls

Ingredients:
Hamburger meat
Soy cheese (not dairy)
Garlic powder
Sweet paprika

Preparation:
Prepare hamburgers (see recipe on page 89).

Break off small amounts to shape into balls twice the size of large olives.

Place the balls on a greased pan and bake in a 180C oven for 30 minutes.

When ready, remove from oven.

Place a piece of soy cheese on each ball and sprinkle with a dash of garlic powder and a dash of paprika.

Return to oven till the cheese has melted.

Remove from oven, place a toothpick into each ball, and serve.

Cherry Tomatoes Stuffed with Chicken Livers

Ingredients:
Chicken livers
Cherry tomatoes

Preparation:
Broil chicken livers till they are cooked in the middle.
Cut into bite-sized pieces.
Cut the tops off the cherry tomatoes.
Stuff each tomato with a piece of chicken liver.
Sprinkle with salt and pepper.
Serve hot or cold.

Tuna on Kohlrabi

Ingredients:
1 can tuna in water (white tuna is best)
fresh kohlrabi
1 teaspoon mustard
1 tablespoon mayonnaise
a red pepper
an onion

Preparation:
Mash the tuna.
Dice the onion finely and add to tuna.
Add mustard and mayonnaise.
Mix till well blended.
Slice the kohlrabi.
Spoon tuna on each slice of kohlrabi.
Place a piece of red pepper on the tuna for decoration.

Home-Marinaded Herring

Ingredients:

5 fillets of matjes herring

1 onion

1 tablespoons vinegar

1 tablespoon fructose

1 bayleaf

1 teaspoon olive oil

Preparation:

Choose even slices of matjes herring.

Cut into bite-sized pieces.

Thinly slice the onion and add.

Add the remaining ingredients.

Mix to blend.

Store in a glass container in the fridge.

Can be eaten after marinating for one day.

Serve on a whole-wheat or rye cracker or trimmed and quartered toast.

Chopped Egg *(with tofu)*

Ingredients:

6 eggs

3 level teaspoons tofu (dig the spoon into the block of tofu to get the required amount)

2 stalks celery

3 tablespoons mayonnaise

1 onion

salt and pepper to taste

Preparation:

Boil eggs till hard.

Cool and dice.

Mash the tofu to the same consistency as the diced egg. Add to egg.

Cut celery lengthwise along the stalk and slice.

Finely dice the onion.

Add remaining ingredients and mix.

Place one thin slice of tomato on a whole-wheat cracker and spoon chopped egg on top.

health. Now you can know what to expect, and this will help prepare you to overcome the irritations that accompany transition and change.

The second category of obstacles is concerned with taste. We have become accustomed to the taste of sweetness in countless ways, most of them unconsciously, and all of them inadvertently. Our palates have become conditioned to the taste of sweet without actively seeking to include sweets in our diet. It wouldn't take a wild imagination to conclude that we have become victims of a sinister plot to instill in us a longing for the taste of sweetness. Many processed foods that are savoury have had sugar added to enhance the taste. Whether sugar is used as a flavor enhancer or as a simple food that stimulates the body to process the glucose, our metabolism has been forced to deal with too much glucose for too long. It may not be a plot, but the damage, for many of us, is an actual addiction, and that is a sinister result.

We aren't aware of the sugar content that is found in almost every processed food we eat. How many people are aware of the sugar content in hamburgers, processed meat, prepared herring, breads, processed soups, burger buns, granola/muesli, and more? This list is longer than we have room for. What's more, when trying to detect which foods contain sugar when we are out shopping for food, only the sharp shoppers among us would know how to go about it. Most of us see a blurb on a package that says the item is sugar-free, and assume that it's a safe bet. Wrong. Another look may reveal that the item contains maltose or honey or some other natural sweetener. In other words, what is apparent at first sight is not necessarily what we expect. As mentioned earlier, the list of ingredients must be thoroughly checked for other sources of glucose, such as dextrose, etc.

This second set of obstacles provides an upside as well as a downside. On the downside, an addiction is a grueling challenge that is always present in the form of a constant, gnawing, incessant demand. It is not easy to give up foods that are addictive. We try and try, but the addiction overcomes us, and we slip back into the mode we tried to escape. We suffer defeat, along with the organic battering that it means physically.

The upside comes from the new coping mechanism that has now become available to you. Unlike the past, when there seemed to be no escape, the "new nutrition" offers you the ability to handle the nagging demand for high-G.I. foods. You can depend on the effects of eating low-fat protein to work for you. Feeling full is the most effective weapon you have at your disposal in your battle against eating the wrong food. Feeling full grants you the moment of sanity that you need when having to make a decision about what should be passing your lips. The more low-fat protein you eat, the more satisfied you'll feel, and the less tempted you'll be to go astray. The preference for sweet and high-G.I. food will start to decline as you eat less of those items. It is actually a reversal of the past when the more you ate, the more you wanted to eat. You'll soon find that the less sweet and starch you eat, the less you need them.

The most gratifying elements in the biochemical process are: it is predictable, it brings fast results, and it is in your control. The addiction to sugar and foods that turn to sugar is an obstacle that has been standing between you and your wish for change.

But it is an addiction that can be harnessed. You're likely to find that the most astonishing aspect of trying to break the high-G.I. habit is the step you have to take to make the decision. That in itself presents more of a challenge than sticking to the decision!

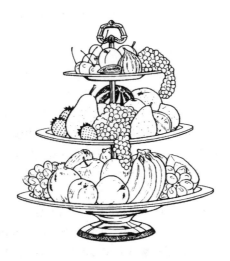

Afterword

Let's look at the list of my symptoms before following the Biochemical Key method. With the explanation of how food groups affect our metabolism, now the puzzle is solved, and we can understand clearly why the symptoms appeared, and why they disappeared!

I had: swelling
Reason: Excess insulin caused the retention of salt and fluid, making my face and legs puffy.

I had: constipation
Reason: In many cases sugar is binding, which firmly condenses the stool.

I had: high blood pressure
Reason: Excess insulin was thickening the artery walls, making it more difficult for the heart to pump.

I had: a craving for chocolate, potato and pasta.
Reason: I was carb-addicted. Eating high G.I. carbs caused a craving for more carbs that was generated by too much insulin in my system.

I had: poor nutrition
Reason: I ate one meal a day to keep my weight down, which did not provide me with adequate nutrition. I now eat three full meals daily. I lost all my excess weight, and the threat of gaining weight has vanished.

I had: morning moodiness

Reason: After high insulin levels during the day, my blood sugar would swing way down after not eating all night. The low blood sugar would cause my irritability.

I had: I didn't feel hungry until I started to eat.

Reason: Once the insulin started to flow, it brought on hunger.

Eat well to feel well and look well!

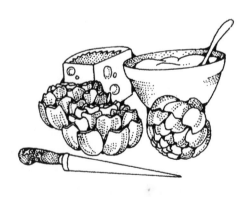